the **Gi** DIET

Shopping and Eating Out Pocket Guide

Rick Gallop

This edition first published in Great Britain in 2005 by
Virgin Books Ltd
Thames Wharf Studios
Rainville Road
London
W6 9HA

First published in 2004

A catalogue record for the book is available from the British Library

ISBN: 0 7535 1032 4

Designed by Smith & Gilmour, London
Printed in the UK by Bath Press, CPI Group

CONTENTS

Introduction

Congratulations! The fact that you're reading this means that you have decided to go on the G.I. Diet – the easiest, healthiest, most effective route to permanent weight loss. Whether you've been losing weight on the plan for a while or are just about to embark on it, *The G.I. Diet Guide to Shopping and Eating Out* will not only make following the programme easier, but will show you how much fun you can have while losing weight. Being on the G.I. Diet doesn't mean that you have to change your lifestyle radically; it was designed with the real world in mind, so that you can eat out, travel, celebrate special events, snack and still lose those extra unwanted pounds. No matter where you go or what the occasion, there are always delicious green-light options to enjoy and the purpose of this book is to list them for you.

The G.I.Diet Guide to Shopping and Eating Out was first published in 2004 and it is intended to be complementary to *The G.I.Diet* and/or *Living the G.I.Diet* and not a replacement for either of those two books, since it doesn't explain the principles of the diet or how it works and without reading and understanding those, this guide will make little sense. So if this book is your first introduction to the G.I.Diet, then I suggest you purchase either *The G.I. Diet* or its companion recipe book *Living the G.I. Diet*.

As in the first edition of this book, *The G.I. Diet Pocket Guide to Shopping and Eating Out* is divided into two main sections. Now more comprehensive in scope and with further information on a variety of areas, Part One, 'At the Supermarket', takes you aisle by aisle through the shop. While the food guides in *The G.I. Diet* and *Living the G.I. Diet* are organised by meal or food group, this guide is organised the way a typical supermarket might be, starting with the fresh produce and ending with frozen foods. You can start at the beginning and let the book navigate your shopping trolley through the supermarket aisles, or you can look up a specific food in the index.

Part Two, 'Eating Out', lists the green-light options available at a number of popular fast food chains and also gives some helpful guidelines to follow when dining out. It lists the dishes you'd typically find at Italian, Greek, Chinese, Indian, Mexican, Thai and Japanese restaurants and points out the green-light options. Eating out should be a fun, social occasion and this guide will help you enjoy it without worrying about your waistline.

One of the popular features of the G.I. Diet is that you don't have to count calories, add points or measure carbs in order to follow it. I've been researching glycemic ratings, fat and calorie levels and ingredient lists of food products and menu items and have done all the maths for you. Now all you have to do is look at the colour-coded charts to find out which foods you can fill your shopping trolley with or order in a restaurant. Although I've included the red- and yellow-light columns along with the green-light, this book is really about the green-light, about all the foods you can enjoy while slimming down.

This diet isn't about deprivation and going hungry: it's about making the right choices and eating until you're satisfied. Food is one of life's greatest pleasures and you can definitely indulge in it. Enjoy!

As always, your feedback is extremely valuable so others can benefit from your experience. I can be reached through my website, at **www.gidiet.com**.

Part One: At the Supermarket

Following the G.I. Diet really begins once you clear out your cupboards and refrigerator of red-light products and make a trip to the supermarket to stock up on green-light ones. A word of advice: don't go to the supermarket until after you've eaten a meal. One of the worst mistakes you can make is to go food shopping on an empty stomach – you'll only feel tempted by all those red-light ready-to-eat foods. You may also want to do a bit of planning before you go. Check out the recipe sections in the revised edition of *The G.I. Diet* and *Living the G.I. Diet*, choose a few that appeal to you and make a list of the ingredients you'll need. Then take it and this guide along with you to the shop. With these tools in hand, you'll find it easy to load your trolley with delicious food and I hope you'll be introduced to some new favourites.

HOW TO USE THIS GUIDE

I've organised the food in this guide the way you would typically find it in the supermarket, in sections such as the Fruit and Vegetable Aisle, the Deli counter, the Bakery, the Meat Counter, the Beverages Aisle, the Frozen Food Section and so on. Within each of these sections you'll find categories of food such as processed meat, breads etc. All are listed in one of the three traffic-light-based colour columns.

If you find a food in the red-light column that you would normally add to your shopping trolley, look at what's listed beside it in the green-light column. There is almost always a wonderful green-light alternative to a red- or yellow-light food. If, for example, you would normally buy a cantaloupe melon, which is a red-light food, choose some peaches or oranges or grapes, or any of the other green-light choices instead. Remember that if you want to look up a specific food rather than a whole category, you can look at the index on page 92.

9

I've generally tried to stay away from listing specific brands. There are just too many out there and they vary from region to region. For the most part they don't have any bearing on the G.I. rating of a particular food anyway. For example, low-fat cottage cheese (1 per cent), or wholemeal spaghetti, or Dijon mustard is pretty much the same no matter who's made it. The only times I have mentioned brands is when it does make a difference. For example, most cereals are red light, but traditional oatmeal is a green-light product.

It can be a bit tricky sometimes distinguishing the green-light products from the red-light. Take bread for example. We know that white bread is red light, since it spikes glucose levels in your bloodstream, releasing insulin, which stores the glucose as fat. The green-light alternative is wholegrain bread, but many of the healthy-looking seven-grain loaves out there are not exactly what they seem. Some of them list 'enriched white flour' or 'unbleached flour' in the ingredients list and this puts a red flashing

light over them. The first ingredient listed on bread should always be '100% wholemeal flour' or '100% wholegrain flour'. If 'stoneground' is mentioned, even better. So checking ingredients lists and labels can be important, and I'll give you some guidelines to follow.

READING LABELS

NUTRITION INFORMATION
TYPICAL VALUES PER ½ PACKET

Energy 1237kJ/298kcal
Protein 8.9g, Carbohydrate
17.5g, of which sugars 4.2g,
Fat 21.3g, of which saturates
4.4g, Fibre 1.6g, Sodium 0.1g.

TYPICAL VALUES PER 100G

Energy 2474kJ/595kcal
Protein 17.8g, Carbohydrate
35.0g, of which sugars 8.4g,
Fat 42.6g, of which saturates
8.8g, Fibre 3.2g, Sodium 0.2g.

1. Serving size

Is this realistic, or is the manufacturer lowering it (often the case with cereals) so the calorie and fat totals in particular look better than the competition? When comparing one brand with another, make sure you are comparing the same serving sizes.

2. Calories

The product with the least amount of calories is obviously the best choice.

3. Fat

Choose the product with the least amount of fat, particularly saturated (bad) fat and avoid any product that contains trans fat – the worst of the saturated fats.

4. Protein

The higher the protein level the better. Protein acts as a brake on the digestive system lowering the G.I. rating of the food.

5. Fibre

The product with the higher fibre content is the best choice, whether it's soluble or insoluble. Fibre, like protein, significantly lowers the G.I. rating.

6. Sugar

Try to avoid products that contain added sugar. Choose the ones with sugar substitutes or none at all. 'Non-fat' products that contain added sugar aren't non-fattening.

7. Sodium (salt)

Look for lower sodium levels. Sodium increases water retention, which causes bloating, added weight and has an adverse effect on blood pressure.

> **TO SUM UP:**
> The best green-light buy is
> • Lower in calories
> • Lower in fat, particularly saturated fat
> • Higher in fibre
> • Lower in sugar and sodium

The Green-Light Shopping Guide

THE FRUIT AND VEGETABLE AISLE

Vegetables and fruit are the cornerstone of the G.I. Diet. They are low G.I. and high in fibre, nutrients, vitamins and minerals. Cooking them raises their G.I. and reduces their nutrient content, so use as little water as possible and cook only until they are just tender – or try eating them raw.

Soya-based foods such as tofu are high in protein, low in saturated fat and good for a healthy heart. Many supermarkets carry something known as Textured Vegetable Protein (TVP) and it is used to make veggie burgers or breakfast sausages and other products. It's an excellent choice whether you're vegetarian or not. Quorn is also a popular alternative.

You can often find nuts and dried fruit in the produce section of the supermarket, or they may be in the home baking section. Most dried fruit is very high in sugar and therefore red light.

However, there are some yellow-light choices, and all dried fruit can be used in modest quantities in baking.

Nuts are an excellent source of good fats and protein and green-light nuts contain even more monounsaturated (best) fat than the others. Remember, though, that all nuts are calorie dense and so must be eaten in limited quantities, about eight to twelve per serving. It's just too easy to unconsciously consume a whole bowl of nuts while watching television, but this quantity would equal your total calorie needs for an entire day!

VEGETABLES
Broad beans
Parsnips
Plantains
Potatoes
(mashed or baked)
Swede
Turnip

VEGETABLES
Artichokes
Beetroot
Corn
Potatoes (boiled)
Pumpkin
Squash
Sweet potatoes
Yams

VEGETABLES
Alfalfa sprouts
Asparagus
Aubergines
Beans
(green/runner)
Bok choy
Broccoli
Brussels sprouts
Cabbage
(all varieties)
Carrots
Cauliflower
Celeriac
Celery
Collard greens
Courgettes
Cucumbers
Edamame
(soya beans)
Endive
Escarole
Fresh herbs
Garlic
Horseradish
Kale
Kohl rabi

Leeks
Lettuce
(all varieties)
Mangetout
Mushrooms
(all varieties)
Mustard greens
New potatoes
Okra
Onions
Peas
Peppers
(sweet or hot)
Raddichio
Radishes
Rocket
Root ginger
Shallots
Spinach
Spring onions
Sugar snap peas
Sun-dried tomatoes
Swiss chard
Tomatoes
Watercress

SOYA/MEAT SUBSTITUTES
Soya cheese
Tofu

SOYA/MEAT SUBSTITUTES
Quorn
Soya cheese (low fat)
TVP products
Tofu (low fat)

FRESH FRUIT
Cantaloupe melon
Honeydew melon
Watermelon

FRESH FRUIT
Apricots
Bananas
Coconut
Custard apples
Kiwi
Mango
Papaya
Passionfruit
Pineapple
Pomegranates

FRESH FRUIT
Apples
Avocado
Blackberries
Cherries
Clementines
Cranberries
Grapefruit
Grapes
Guavas
Lemons
Mandarin oranges
Nectarines
Oranges
Peaches
Pears
Plums
Raspberries
Rhubarb
Strawberries
Tangerines

NUTS
Chocolate-
covered nuts

NUTS
Brazil nuts
Peanuts
Pecans
Walnuts

NUTS
Almonds
Cashews
Hazelnuts
Macadamias
Pistachios

DRIED FRUIT
Dates
Dried mango
Dried papaya
Dried pineapple
Figs
Raisins

DRIED FRUIT
Dried apricots
Dried cranberries
Prunes

DRIED FRUIT
Dried apples

THE DELI COUNTER

Most processed meats are high in fat, sodium and sodium nitrates and are therefore red light. There are, however, a few yellow- and green-light options. Cheese, too, is pretty much a diet villain, since it's high in saturated fats. However, for flavour it can be used sparingly, sprinkled on salads, omelettes and pasta.

PROCESSED MEAT
Bologna
Hot dogs
Liverwurst
Pancetta
Pastrami (beef)
Pâté
Roast beef
Salami
Sausage
Smoked meat

PROCESSED MEAT
Corned beef

PROCESSED MEAT
Chicken breast
Lean ham
Turkey breast
Turkey roll

CHEESE
Most cheese

CHEESE
Low-fat cheese

CHEESE
Extra low-fat cheese
(e.g. Laughing Cow
Light, Boursin Light)
Fat-free cheese

OTHER
Blue cheese dip
Butternut
squash dip
Coleslaw
Pasta salads
Polenta
Tuna salad
Tzatziki

OTHER
Baba ghanouj

OTHER
Olives
Hummus
Roasted red
pepper dip

THE BAKERY

Anything that is made primarily of bleached white flour – which has one of the highest G.I. ratings of any food – is red light. Because most people are in the habit of eating white bread, which has been stripped of most of its nutrients, they are unused to wholegrain breads. But once you give them a chance, I think you'll find green-light breads far more flavourful than bland white loaves.

Always check labels when choosing a loaf. The first ingredient should be 100 per cent wholemeal or wholegrain flour, and there should be a minimum of 2.5 to 3.0 grams of fibre per slice.

While all the desserts you'll find in the bakery section are red light because of the white flour and sugar in them, you can make your own delectable desserts at home, using the recipes in *The G.I. Diet* or *Living the G.I. Diet*.

BREAD

Bagels
Baguette
Breadcrumbs
Cornbread
Croissants
Croutons
Crumpets
Flatbread
Hamburger buns
Hot dog buns
Ice cream cones
Kaiser rolls
Muffins (flat
and American)
Pitta
Raisin bread
Stuffing
Tortillas
White bread

BREAD

Crispbreads
with fibre
Pitta (wholemeal)
Pumpernickel
Rye
Sourdough
Thin wholemeal
Pizza crust
Tortillas
(wholemeal)
Wholegrain breads

BREAD

100% stoneground
wholemeal bread
Crispbreads with
high fibre
Wholegrain,
high-fibre breads
(2.5–3.0g fibre
per slice)

THE FISH COUNTER

All fish and shellfish are green light and provide
a wide variety of wonderful meals. Some people
are under the mistaken belief that oily fish,
such as salmon and mackerel, isn't good for you.
In fact, oily fish is rich in omega-3 and is therefore
extremely beneficial for heart health.

FISH
All breaded fish
Breaded calamari
Fish tinned in oil
Sushi

FISH
Salt cod

FISH
All fresh fish
All frozen fish
Caviar
Fish tinned
in water
Pickled herring
Sashimi
Smoked fish
Squid

SHELLFISH
Breaded clams
Breaded scallops
Breaded
prawns/scampi
Seafood pâté

SHELLFISH
Seafood salads

SHELLFISH
Tinned clams
Tinned crab
Tinned lobster
Tinned prawns
Fresh clams
Fresh crab
Imitation crab
Lobster
Mussels
Oysters
Prawns
Scallops
Scampi
Smoked oysters

THE MEAT COUNTER

Meat always contains some fat, but some cuts have far less than others. Simply trimming visible fat can reduce the overall amount by an average of 50 per cent. Remember to keep the serving size to 4 ounces, which is about the size of the palm of your hand.

Skinless chicken or turkey breast is really the benchmark for low-fat protein. Dark meat, or thighs and legs, duck and goose are higher in saturated fat.

BEEF
Beef steaks
on the bone
Brisket
Minced beef
Sausages
T-bone steak

PORK
Chops on the bone
Blade
Sausages
Spare ribs
Streaky bacon

**CHICKEN, GAME
& TURKEY**
Breast with skin
Roasted
chicken/casseroled
light/dark with skin
Thigh with skin
Wing with skin

BEEF
Beef jerky
Corned beef
Fillet
Lean mince
Sirloin

PORK
Centre loin
Fresh ham
Shank
Sirloin
Top loin

**CHICKEN, GAME
& TURKEY**
Roasted/casseroled
light/dark without skin
Thigh without skin
Turkey bacon
Turkey sausage

BEEF
Extra lean mince
Tournedos

PORK
Back bacon
Fillet
Lean deli ham
Tenderloin

**CHICKEN, GAME
& TURKEY**
Breast without skin

VEAL
Breaded escalope
Sausages

LAMB
Rack
Sausages

DUCK & GOOSE
Duck (all parts)
Goose (all parts)

OTHER
Offal
Organ meat

LAMB
Fore shank
Leg shank
Loin chop

VEAL
Chops on the bone
Cutlets
Loin chop
Rib roast
Shank

OTHER
Elk
Emu
Hare
Rabbit
Ostrich
Venison

THE TINNED BEANS
AND VEGETABLE AISLE

Beans, or legumes, are the perfect green-light food. They are rich in protein and fibre and low in fat. Tinned beans are more convenient than dried beans, but the canning process significantly raises their G.I. rating – sometimes up to 50 per cent. Likewise, with vegetables. It is always preferable to buy fresh or frozen vegetables rather than tinned.

DRIED BEANS
Black beans
Black-eyed peas
Butter beans
Chickpeas
Haricots
Kidney beans
Lentils
Mung
Soyabeans
Split peas

TINNED BEANS
Baked beans
with sausages
Broad
Refried

TINNED BEANS
Baked beans
Chilli

TINNED BEANS
Baked beans
(low fat)
Black beans
Black-eyed peas
Butter beans
Chick peas
Haricots
Lentils
Mung
Pigeon
Soyabeans

TINNED AND BOTTLED VEGETABLES
Artichoke hearts
Creamed corn
Beetroot
Peas
Potatoes
Sweet potatoes
Yams

TINNED AND BOTTLED VEGETABLES
Most tinned vegetables
Sun-dried tomatoes in oil

TINNED AND BOTTLED VEGETABLES
Roasted red peppers
Tinned tomatoes
Tomato Puree

THE PASTA AND SAUCES AISLE

Most pasta is green light, and wholemeal pasta is even more so. Make sure that you always slightly undercook pasta – until it's just *al dente*, as the Italians say – and watch the serving size (75-100g [3–4oz] per serving).

Choose low-sugar pasta sauces made primarily of tomatoes. Tomato sauce happens to be rich in lycoprene, which has been shown to reduce the risk of prostate cancer. Sauces with cream and/or cheese are, of course, red light.

PASTA
All tinned pasta
Gnocchi
Macaroni cheese
Noodles (tinned
or instant)
Pasta filled with
cheese or meat

PASTA
Rice noodles

PASTA
Capellini
Fettuccine
Linguine
Macaroni
Penne
Rigatoni
Spaghetti
Vermicelli

PASTA SAUCES
Cream sauces
Sauces with added
meat or cheese
Sauces with added
sugar or sucrose

PASTA SAUCES
Basil pesto
Sauces with vegetables
(no added sugar)

PASTA SAUCES
Healthy Choice
pasta sauces
Light sauces
with vegetables
(no added sugar)

THE SOUP, TINNED SEAFOOD, MEAT AND POULTRY AISLE

Tinned soups generally have a higher G.I. rating than soups made from scratch because of the high processing temperatures needed to prevent spoilage. So if you have the time, it's worthwhile to make your own with green-light ingredients. The best tinned soups are the ones that are vegetable based, are not pureed and don't contain cream.

SOUP
All cream-
based soups
Tinned black bean
Tinned puréed
vegetable
Tinned split pea
Instant soups

TINNED SEAFOOD
Fish tinned in oil

TINNED MEAT
Beef
Ham
Pork
Spam

SOUP
Tinned chicken
noodle
Tinned lentil
Tinned tomato

TINNED MEAT
Chicken
Turkey

SOUP
Baxter's Healthy
Choice
Bouillon
(low sodium)
Tinned low-fat bean
and vegetable soups
Miso soup

TINNED SEAFOOD
Fish tinned in water
Crab
Prawns
Smoked oysters

THE GRAINS AND SIDE DISHES AISLE

Whole grains with all the nutrition and fibre intact are usually green light. With rice, it all depends on the variety, because some contain a starch, amylase, that breaks down slowly.

GRAINS

Amaranth
Arborio rice
Couscous
Grits
Instant rice
Jasmine rice
Millet
Rice
Semolina
Short-grain rice
Sticky rice

SIDE DISHES

Instant noodles
Instant potatoes
Stuffing

GRAINS

Cornmeal
Kamut
Kasha
Spelt

GRAINS

Barley
Basmati rice
Brown rice
Buckwheat
Bulgur
Flax seeds
Long-grain rice
Quinoa
Wheat berries
Wild rice

THE INTERNATIONAL FOODS AISLE

ASIAN
Tinned lychees
in syrup
Chow mein noodles
Chutney
Coconut milk
Ghee
Honey garlic sauce
Instant noodles
Plum sauce
Ramen noodles
Sweet and
sour sauce

ASIAN
Black bean sauce
Tinned baby corn
Tinned lychees in juice
Coconut milk (light)
Fish sauce (nam pla)
Oyster sauce
Pappadums (baked)
Rice noodles
Rice wine
Sesame oil
Soy sauce (regular)
Udon noodles

ASIAN
Buckwheat noodles
Tinned bamboo
shoots
Tinned water
chestnuts
Cellophane
(mung bean) noodles
Chilli sauce
Curry paste
Dried seaweed
Hoisin sauce
Hot chilli paste
Miso
Pickled ginger
Rice Vinegar
Soy sauce
(low sodium)
Teriyaki sauce
Vermicelli
Wasabi

MEXICAN
Refried beans
Taco shells
Tortillas
Tostades

MEXICAN
Salsa (with
added sugar)
Taco sauce
(with added sugar)

MEXICAN
Tinned green chillis
Chipotle en adobo
Pickled jalapenos
Salsa (with no
added sugar)
Taco sauce (with
no added sugar)

MIDDLE EASTERN
Couscous
Pitta bread
Stuffed vine leaves

MIDDLE EASTERN
Baba ghanouj
Wholemeal
pitta bread

MIDDLE EASTERN
Falafel mix
Hummus
Tahini

THE COOKING OIL, VINEGAR, SALAD DRESSING AND PICKLES AISLE

Choosing the right oil to use in cooking and on salads is critical to the health of your heart. Saturated and hydrogenated oils are dangerous and should be avoided. Canola (rapeseed) and olive oils get the green light.

Because acid tends to reduce the G.I. rating of a meal – it slows the digestive process – vinegars and vinaigrettes are great additions. Dressings should always be low fat, but be careful of sugar levels. Sometimes producers will raise the sugar level as they reduce the oil to improve flavour. Be sure to check labels and compare low-fat brands.

COOKING OIL
Coconut oil
Palm oil
Vegetable-based
margarines

COOKING OIL
Corn oil
Peanut oil
Sesame oil
Soya oil
Sunflower oil
Vegetable oil

COOKING OIL
Canola oil
Extra-virgin olive oil
Flax oil
Olive oil
Vegetable oil spray

VINEGAR
Balsamic vinegar
Cider vinegar
Red wine vinegar
Rice vinegar
White vinegar
White wine vinegar

SALAD DRESSINGS
Regular salad
dressings

SALAD DRESSINGS
Light salad
dressings

SALAD DRESSINGS
Low-fat, low-sugar
salad dressings
Low-fat, low-sugar
vinaigrettes

PICKLES

Branston pickle
Chutney
Gherkins
Piccalilli
Pickled beetroot
Sweet mustard
pickles

PICKLES

Sun-dried
tomatoes in oil

PICKLES

Capers
Cocktail onions
Dill pickles
Olives
Pickled hot peppers
Pickled mixed
vegetables
Pickled mushrooms
Sauerkraut

CONDIMENTS

Barbecue sauce
Honey mustard
Ketchup
Mayonnaise
Relish
Tartar sauce

CONDIMENTS

Hot sauce
Salsa

CONDIMENTS

Chilli sauce
Dijon mustard
Gravy mix (maximum
20 calories per 120ml
[4fl oz] serving)
Horseradish
Mayonnaise (fat free)
Mustard
Salsa
(no added sugar)
Seafood
cocktail sauce
Steak sauce
Tabasco
Worcestershire sauce

THE SNACKS AISLE

Unfortunately, the snacks aisle at the supermarket is full of red-light temptation. Still, all you G.I. dieters need three snacks a day – green-light ones of course. If you buy food bars, make sure they contain 20–30 g of carbohydrates, 12–15 g of protein and 5 g of fat. A good green-light choice is Slim Fast (half a bar per serving).

SNACKS

Caramel-coated popcorn
Cheese puffs
Crackers
Flavoured gelatine (all varieties)
Fruit chews
Granola bars
Ice cream cones
Melba toast
Party mix
Popcorn (regular)
Pretzels
Pudding
Rice cakes
Rice crackers
Rice crisps
Sweets
Tortilla chips
Trail mix

SNACKS

Dark chocolate (70% cocoa)
Most nuts
Popcorn (air popped)
Roasted peanuts
Salsa (with added sugar)

SNACKS

Almonds
Applesauce (unsweetened)
Cashews
Food bars
Fruit bowls with no added sugar
Hazelnuts
Macadamia nuts
Pistachios
Pumpkin seeds
Salsa (with no added sugar)
Soyanuts
Sugar-free boiled sweets
Sunflower seeds
Tinned fruit salad
Tinned mandarin oranges
Tinned peaches in juice or water
Tinned pears in juice or water

THE BAKING AISLE

Though you can't eat ready-made baked goods from the supermarket when you're trying to lose weight, you can bake your own sweet treats using recipes from *The G.I. Diet* and *Living the G.I. Diet*. They call for sugar substitutes rather than sugar, honey or treacle. Our favourite brand of sweetener is Splenda, which is derived from sugar but doesn't have the calories. A small amount of dried fruit is acceptable for baking.

SWEETENERS
Corn syrup
Glucose
Honey
Molasses
Sugar (all types)
Treacle

SWEETENERS
Fructose

SWEETENERS
Aspartame
Hermesetas Gold
Splenda
Stevia
Sweet 'N Low

**SPICES AND
FLAVOURINGS**
Coating for
poultry or pork

**SPICES AND
FLAVOURINGS**
Bouillon
Bovril
Marmite

**SPICES AND
FLAVOURINGS**
Bouillon
(low sodium)
Herbs
Extracts (vanilla etc)
Gravy mixes
(20 calories
maximum per 120ml
[4fl oz] serving)
Lemon juice
Lime juice
Pepper
Salt
Seasoning mixes
with no added sugar
Spices

BAKING SUPPLIES

Biscuit mixes
Cake mixes
Cranberry sauce
(tinned)
Chocolate chips
Evaporated milk
Glacé cherries
Graham cracker
crumbs
Icing
Lard
Maraschino
cherries
Mincemeat
Muffin mixes
Peanut butter
(regular and light)
Pie filling
Raisins
Sweetened
condensed milk
Vegetable fat
White flour

BAKING SUPPLIES

Baking chocolate
(unsweetened)
Coconut
Dried apricots
Dried cranberries
Natural nut
butters
Peanuts
Pecans
Pine nuts
Prunes
Walnuts

BAKING SUPPLIES

Almonds
Baking powder
Cashews
Cocoa
Hazelnuts
Macadamia nuts
Oat bran
Pumpkin seeds
Sunflower seeds
Wheat bran
Wheat germ
Wholemeal flour

CEREALS AND BREAKFAST FOODS AISLE

Of course, the king of breakfast foods is old-fashioned oatmeal – the large flake kind, not instant or quick oats. Most cereals on the market are red light as they're made from highly processed grains that lack both nutrition and fibre. Beware of those so-called healthy or natural granola-types of cereal, because, they, too, are usually low in fibre and high in sugar. What you should be looking for are cereals that have at least 10 grams of fibre per serving. They can be dressed up with nuts, fruit and yoghurt. Cereal bars are absolutely red light – they're full of sugar. Better to go for a Slim Fast bar. While packaged pancake mixes and frozen waffles are red light, you can make green-light versions yourself (the recipes are in *Living the G.I. Diet*).

Low-sugar fruit spreads or jams that list fruit as the first ingredient are wonderful green-light additions to toast, cereal and low-fat dairy products such as yoghurt and cottage cheese.

CEREAL
All cereals
except those
listed as yellow
or green light
Cereal bars
Cream of wheat
Granola
Instant porridge
Muesli
Quick-cooking
oatmeal

PANCAKES
AND SYRUPS
Corn syrup
Maple syrup
Molasses
Pancake mix
Pancake syrup
Treacle

CEREAL
Shredded
wheat bran

CEREAL
100% bran
All-Bran
Bran Buds
Fibre 1
Fibre First
Large-flake
oatmeal
Oat bran
Steel-cut
Irish oatmeal

SPREADS AND JAMS
Fruit spreads
(regular)
Jam
Marmalade
Nutella
Peanut butter
(regular and light)

SPREADS AND JAMS
Natural nut
butters
Natural peanut
butter

SPREADS AND JAMS
Fruit spreads/Jams
(extra fruit, no
added sugar)

THE BEVERAGES AISLE

You need up to eight glasses of liquid a day
to keep your body hydrated and healthy. Drinks
with caffeine tend to stimulate the appetite and
so are red light. The exception is tea, which has
far less caffeine than either coffee or soft drinks.
Juice is not worth the calories – eat the fruit
instead. In addition to the green-light beverages
listed on page 52 remember that skimmed milk
and light, plain soya milk , which are found
in the dairy section, also make refreshing and
nutritious drinks.

BEVERAGES

Chocolate milk mix
Coffee (regular)
Coffee whitener
Evaporated milk
Fruit crystals
Fruit drinks
Hot chocolate
(regular)
Iced tea (regular)
Soft drinks
(regular)
Sports drinks
Sweetened
condensed milk
Sweetened juice
Tonic water
Watermelon juice

BEVERAGES

Diet soft drinks
(caffeinated)
Most unsweetened
juice
Non-alcoholic beer
Vegetable juices

BEVERAGES

Bottled water
(sparkling or still)
Decaffeinated
coffee
Diet soft drinks
(without caffeine)
Herbal teas
Iced tea (with
no added sugar)
Light instant
chocolate
Tea (with or
without caffeine)

THE DAIRY CABINET

Low-fat dairy products are a G.I. Diet staple.
They're rich in protein, calcium and vitamin D.
Regular dairy products contain a high amount
of saturated fat and are therefore red light. But
you can lightly sprinkle full-flavoured cheeses
such as mature cheddar, feta and Parmesan over
salads, omelettes and pasta. If you are lactose
intolerant, low-fat soya products are an excellent
alternative – just make sure they aren't laden
with sugar.

You may often find a selection of non-dairy
products in the dairy cabinet, too, such as
pickles, biscuit mix and anchovy paste, which I
have also listed.

MILK
Almond milk
Chocolate milk
Cream
Goat milk
Regular soya milk
Rice milk
Whole or
2% fat milk

CHEESE
Cheese (regular)
Cheese spread
Cottage cheese
(whole or 2% fat)
Cream cheese

**YOGHURT AND
SOUR CREAM**
Sour cream
Yoghurt
(whole or 2% fat)

MILK
1% fat milk

CHEESE
Cheese (low-fat)
Low-fat
cream cheese
Low-fat mozzarella
Regular soya
cheese

**YOGHURT AND
SOUR CREAM**
Sour cream (light)
Yoghurt (low-fat,
with sugar)

MILK
Buttermilk
Skimmed milk
Soya milk
(plain, low-fat)

CHEESE
Cheese (fat-free)
Cottage cheese
(1% or fat-free)
Extra low-fat cheese
(e.g., Laughing Cow
Light, Boursin Light)
Low-fat soya cheese

**YOGHURT AND
SOUR CREAM**
Fruit yoghurt
(non-fat with
sugar substitute)
Sour cream (non-fat)

BUTTER AND MARGARINE
Butter
Hard margarine

EGGS
Whole,
regular eggs

OTHER
Biscuit dough
Dips
Eggnog
Flavoured gelatine
Pickled eggs
Readymade pastry
Suet
Sweetened juice

BUTTER AND MARGARINE
Soft margarine
(nonhydrogenated)

EGGS
Whole omega-3 eggs

OTHER
Anchovy paste
Unsweetened juice

BUTTER AND MARGARINE
Soft margarine
(nonhydrogenated,
light)

EGGS
Egg whites
in cartons
Liquid eggs
in cartons

OTHER
Dill pickles
Gefilte fish
Horseradish
Pickled herrings
Pickled sweet
pimentos
Pickled tomatoes

THE FROZEN FOOD SECTION

Almost all the prepared meals you find in the frozen food section of your supermarket are red light because of the ingredients used and the way in which they've been processed. Still, the freezer section is a great source of green-light convenience foods such as frozen vegetables and fruit, fish and green-light desserts. Make sure the vegetables aren't in a butter, cream or cheese sauce – that's definitely red light!

VEGETABLES
Broad beans
French fries
Hash browns
Lima beans
Swede
Vegetables in a
butter, cream or
cheese sauce

VEGETABLES
Artichoke hearts
Corn
Squash

VEGETABLES
Asparagus
Beans
(green/runner)
Broccoli
Brussels sprouts
Carrots
Cauliflower
Okra
Peas
Peppers
Spinach

PREPARED FOOD

Appetisers
Chicken wings
Dumplings
Lasagne
Meat pies
Pasta filled with
cheese or meat
Pizza
Rice dishes
TV dinners
White bread

BREAKFAST

Hash browns
Sausages
Waffles

PREPARED FOOD

Lean burgers
Pork souvlaki
Soft margarine
(nonhydrogenated)
Turkey burgers

BREAKFAST

Soft margarine
(nonhydrogenated)

PREPARED FOOD

Chicken souvlaki
Extra-lean burgers
Frozen fish without
breaded coating
Quorn
Scallops without
breaded coating
Scampi and prawns
without breaded
coating
Veggie burgers
Textured Vegetable
Protein

DESSERTS

Frozen soya
Desserts (regular)
Ice cream (regular)
Pies
Pie and tart shells
Popsicles
Puff pastry
Tartufo
Whipped topping

DESSERTS

Fruit bars
(no added sugar)

DESSERTS

Frozen soya desserts
with less than
100 calories per
120 g (4oz)
Ice cream (low-fat
and no added sugar)

FRUIT

Blackberries
Blueberries
Cherries
Cranberries
Peaches
Raspberries
Rhubarb
Strawberries

Part Two: Eating Out

FAST FOOD

Just a few years ago the idea of ordering a green-light lunch at a fast food outlet was simply laughable – but no longer! Due in part to the threat of legal action and in part to stagnant market shares, the major fast food chains are finally offering some healthy options. In all fairness, Subway has been pioneering the move towards fast, healthy meals for some time now, and their initiative has been reflected in their phenomenal growth. They have actually replaced McDonald's as North America's number one fast food chain.

Unfortunately, the majority of the food on offer at fast food restaurants is still red light: hamburgers soaked in saturated fat, fish and chicken coated in deep-fried batter, and all the trimmings, such as fries, fizzy drinks, shakes and ketchup, loaded with fat and sugar. To compound this dietary disaster, you can supersize everything!

No wonder we're setting obesity records and becoming diabetics at an exceptional rate.

One of the health issues that is rarely mentioned in the debate on fast food is sodium levels. When creating lower fat products, the fast food industry frequently boosts salt content to make up for any perceived flavour shortfall. The problem is that sodium increases water retention, which causes bloating and extra weight – especially in women – and raises blood pressure. The official recommended daily allowance of sodium is 1,500 milligrams. On average we consume three times that. Though some dishes in some of the fast food chains may appear to be healthy and low in fat, they can have salt levels that are nearly twice what you need for an entire day! In order to alert you to the sodium levels in the fast food I've listed, I've asterisked those items that have excessively high levels, and double-asterisked the ones that reach a stratospheric level.

So what are the points of light in this sea
of gloom? I've listed them by each major fast
food chain. All the items listed are green light.
Remember always to throw away the top half
of the bun on burgers or bread on sandwiches
and eat them open-faced and to ask for low-fat
dressings and use only half the packet on
your salad.

McDonald's

SALADS
Grilled Chicken Caesar Salad (hold the croutons)
Grilled Chicken Ranch Salad

SANDWICHES/BURGERS
Low-fat Grilled Chicken
Grilled Chicken Flat Bread
Quorn Premiere

SNACKS
Oatso Simple + jam
Fruit and yoghurt

Wendy's

SALADS
Mandarin Chicken Salad with roasted almonds.
Spring Mix Salad with roasted pecans

BURGERS
Ultimate Chicken Grilled Sandwich*(open-faced)
plus side salad

DRESSINGS
Fat-free French Style
Reduced Fat Creamy Ranch
Low-fat Honey Mustard

CHILLI
Large Chilli plus side salad with low-fat dressing

SNACKS
Frosty Junior (6oz cup)

Burger King

SALADS
Flame Grilled Chicken Salad
Warmer Crispy Chicken Salad
Premium Caesar Salad

BURGERS/SANDWICHES
Piri Piri Chicken Baguette*
Flame Grilled Chicken Sandwich

DRESSINGS
Honey and mustard
Tomato and basil
French

SNACKS
Twin Pot Bio Yoghurt
Twin Pot Fresh Fruit

Subway

SANDWICHES (6in under 6g fat subs)
Ham*
Honey Mustard Ham*
Roast beef*
Roast chicken breast
Subway Club*
Sweet Onion and Chicken Teriyaki*
Turkey breast*
Turkey Breast, Ham and Roast Beef*
Veggie Delite

DELI SUBS
Ham Deli
Roast Beef Deli
Turkey Breast Deli

SALADS
Garden Fresh (side salad)
Mediterranean Chicken

DRESSINGS
Fat-free Honey Mustard
Fat-free Sweet Onion

WRAPS
Grilled Chicken
Turkey Breast

Prêt a Manger

SANDWICHES
Slim Prêt – Hummus and Tomato
           – Crayfish and Rocket
Fresh Herb Chicken No Mayo
No Bread Tuna Sandwich

SALADS
Ham Salad Mayo Frais
Chicken Salad Mayo Frais
No Bread Chicken Caesar

Other Fast Food Chains

If you go into other fast food outlets, such as
Tesco Express, Sainsbury Local, Marks & Spencer,
Benjys etc, steer clear of sandwiches and rolls
containing mayonnaise and cheese. Look for
wholemeal and high-fibre breads and eat them
open-faced.

NOTE

This information was correct when this guide
went to press. However, as this is a dynamic field,
you may wish to check the websites of fast food
chains from time to time to see if they have
expanded their green-light offerings.

Sandwich Bars

Sandwich Bars are an excellent alternative as they enable you to customise your sandwich and see exactly what is going into it. Here is what to ask for to ensure your sandwich is green light:

• Wholemeal or granary bread

• Hummus or mustard in lieu of butter, margarine or mayonnaise

• Lean slices of chicken or turkey breast, ham or tuna as the principal filling. Avoid mayonnaise, cheese and bacon bits

• Add lots of vegetables such as tomatoes, avocado, lettuce, salad leaves, or onion rings for flavour and nutrition

• Always remove the top slice of bread and eat the sandwich open-faced.

Restaurants

It isn't difficult to eat out the green-light way now that restaurants are following healthy trends such as grilling instead of frying, using vegetable oils and offering a greater variety of fish dishes, vegetables and salads. Here are my top ten tips for ensuring that your night out doesn't leave you feeling guilty the next day:

1. Eat a small bowl of green-light cereal (such as All Bran) with skimmed milk and sweetener just before you leave for the restaurant. This will give you some extra fibre and help take the edge off your appetite .

2. On arrival at the restaurant, drink a glass of water to help you feel a bit fuller. Feel free to enjoy a glass of red wine, but wait until the main course arrives to drink it.

3. Once the habitual basket of rolls or bread – which you ignore – has been passed round the table, ask the waiter to remove it. The longer it sits there, the more tempted you'll be to dig in.

4. Order a chunky vegetable-based soup or a salad with the dressing on the side (no Caesar) to start with, and tell the waiter you would like this as soon as possible.

5. Ask for vegetables instead of potatoes and rice, since you can't be sure of what type will be served.

6. Stick with low-fat cuts of meat or poultry (see page 26), or choose fish or shellfish that isn't breaded or battered. Because restaurant servings tend to be overly generous, remember to eat only 120–175g (4–6oz) – about the size of a pack of cards – and leave the rest.

7. Ask that any sauces that come with your meal be put on the side.

8. Desserts are almost always a dietary minefield with not a lot of green-light choices. Fresh fruit or berries without ice cream is the best option. Or perhaps order a decaffeinated skimmed-milk latte and sweeten it with sugar substitute.

If social pressure to have a rich dessert becomes overwhelming, ask for extra forks so it can be shared. A couple of forkfuls or so with your coffee should get you off the hook with minimal dietary damage!

9. Order only decaffeinated coffee or tea. My favourite choice is a non-fat decaf cappuccino.

10. Finally, and perhaps most importantly, **eat slowly**. The famous Dr Johnson advised chewing food 32 times before swallowing! Although that is a bit over the top, try to put your fork down between mouthfuls. The stomach can take between 20 and 30 minutes to let the brain know it feels full.

ALL-YOU-CAN-EAT BUFFETS

A buffet can be your best or worst option, depending on your self-control. While you're free to make your own selections, there may be a lot of red-light temptations there. I suggest you do a quick reconnaissance of the whole buffet before picking up your plate and starting. This will ensure that there's still space on your plate when you reach your favourite foods. Follow the G.I. Diet ground rules and the buffet will be your best dining-out option bar none.

INTERNATIONAL CUISINE

When eating the same type of food week after week starts to get a bit uninspiring, how about trying something completely new? I love international cuisine, particularly Italian, Greek, Chinese and Indian food. Because we're often unfamiliar with how an exotic dish is made, it's hard to determine whether it's green light or not. In this section I've tried to eliminate some of the guess work by listing the dishes you'd typically find on a menu. Don't hesitate to ask your server about any dish I haven't mentioned. Here's a list of possible requests that could help give your meal a green light:

- Please ask the chef to prepare this dish without a cream sauce.

- Please ask the chef to prepare this dish with the least amount of oil possible.

- Could I order only half a serving of this dish?

- Please replace the potatoes with extra vegetables.

- Could I have the dressing/gravy/sauce on the side?

ITALIAN

If you're serious about sticking to the G.I. Diet, it's really not a good idea to head to a pizzeria. Instead, go to a restaurant that has a wide variety of dishes on the menu. Usually they are divided into a number of parts: *l'antipasto*, which translates as 'before the meal', includes hot and cold appetisers; *il primo*, or 'the first course', which includes pasta, pizza or risotto; *il secondo*, 'the second course' that includes meat, poultry or fish; and *il dolce* is 'dessert'.

Your best bets on the list of antipasti are soups containing beans and vegetables, such as minestrone, and salads, particularly the basic *insalata mista*. Remember to ask for the dressing on the side. Mussels are a good choice provided they are not served in a cream sauce. Other antipasto items such as roasted red peppers or mushrooms sound both delicious and healthy, but be careful of any that are marinated in oil. Although olive oil is beneficial, it is still high in calories. About 240ml (8fl oz) equals the total daily calorie requirement for most people.

Although you should never make a meal of pasta, you can enjoy it as a first course. Choose pasta with a tomato-based sauce and share it with a dinner companion. Your serving should not exceed one quarter of the plate. Avoid pasta stuffed with meat and cheese, pasta in cream sauces and gnocchi. Decline the offer of grated cheese.

If you're craving pizza instead of pasta, choose one with a very thin crust, tomato sauce and vegetable toppings. Ask for no cheese except for a sprinkling of Parmesan. Then have only one slice, sharing the rest with the others at the table, Pizza should also be treated as an appetiser rather than as a meal.

For your *secondo*, choose grilled, roasted or braised fish, chicken or meat. Veal, a mainstay on Italian menus, is low in saturated fat and therefore an excellent choice, unless it is cooked in butter or served with cream sauce.

Watch the serving size – you can always leave some on your plate if necessary. The Italian restaurant I frequent serves a fabulous veal chop, but it is about 14 ounces and comes with mashed potatoes. I ask for extra vegetables instead of the potatoes and share the veal with my wife, Ruth. We also order an extra vegetable or pasta dish to share.

For dessert, I highly recommend a skimmed-milk decaf cappuccino – delicious! You won't miss the highly fattening tiramisu. If you're in a celebratory mood, treat yourself to some *gelato* (ice cream), but since it is high in sugar, split it with a friend.

ITALIAN

Breaded aubergine (or any breaded vegetable)
Fried calamari
Garlic bread
Gnocchi
Mozzarella or bocconcini and tomato salads
Pasta filled with meat or cheese
Pasta with cream or cheese sauce
Risotto
Salads with creamy dressings such as Caesar

ITALIAN

Mussels in wine sauces (no cream)
Roast or braised lamb
Thin-crust pizzas without cheeses

ITALIAN

Grilled fish and chicken
Grilled prawns, scallops or calamari
Grilled, steamed or boiled vegetables
Mussels with tomato sauce (no wine)
Pasta with seafood in tomato sauce (¼ plate only)
Pasta with vegetables in tomato sauce (¼ plate only)
Roasted fish
Veal without cream or butter sauce

GREEK

Greek restaurants often offer a selection of small dishes called *meze*. Two or three of these, such as hummus and grilled calamari can be a meal in themselves when served with small pieces of wholemeal pitta bread and raw vegetables for dipping.

Grilled or baked seafood makes an excellent dinner choice. And the classic chicken souvlaki dinner can be good. Though the serving sizes are often too large, just stick to the recommended green-light servings and you'll be fine. If the rice appears glutinous or sticky avoid it. If potatoes are served with the rice, ask for vegetables instead. A Greek salad often comes with your souvlaki dinner. If this is the case, ask that the feta and dressing be served on the side.

Greek desserts are calorie laden – particularly the ever popular baklava – and thus red light.

GREEK

Baklava
Breaded calamari
Dolmades
Gyros
Kleftiko
Moussaka
Pastitsio
Potato gemistes
Spanakopita
(spinach pie)
Tzatziki

GREEK

Baba ghanouj
Grilled lamb chops
Lamb souvlaki
Pork souvlaki
Vegetable gemista

GREEK

Chicken souvlaki
Grilled or
baked seafood
Hummus
Melitzanosalata
(baked aubergine)

CHINESE

It is a real challenge to eat the green-light way at a Chinese restaurant. Much of the food is deep fried or drowning in sweet sauces and therefore a disaster for your waistline. The sodium levels in the sauces are often very high, and saturated and trans fat oils are sometimes used in cooking. However, it is not impossible to get a green-light meal. Pass on the spring rolls, crispy fried duck, fried rice and dumplings, and look for dishes that contain steamed or stir-fried vegetables with oyster sauce, garlic and ginger. Since many Chinese dishes rest on beds of rice or noodles, you need to pay attention to both type and amount. Most of the rice used is short grain with a glutinous sticky surface and this is red light. Ask if they have long grain or brown rice instead – you may be lucky. Make sure that it is steamed.

Noodles, for the most part, are red light except for 'cellophane noodles', which are made from mung beans. Keep the noodle proportion to no more than one quarter of your plate – it's too easy to heap them up. Stick with savoury sauces and avoid sweet and sour dishes. Try eating with chopsticks – they will slow you down so you end up eating less.

CHINESE
Chinese omelettes
Chow mein
Dumplings
Lo mein
Spring rolls
Sweet and
sour dishes
Wonton soup

CHINESE
Beef in black
bean sauce
Plain noodles
Stir-fried seafood,
chicken or meat
with vegetables
(cooked in a small
amount of oil)

CHINESE
Cellophane noodles
(mung bean noodles)
Hot and sour soup
Sautéed vegetables
with garlic
Steamed seafood
Steamed tofu
with vegetables
Steamed vegetables

INDIAN/SOUTH ASIAN

Vegetables, legumes and basmati rice are predominant in Indian cuisine. Many South Asians are vegetarians whose protein source is lentils and beans. Servings of meat, poultry or fish tend to be modest when used, and all this makes an Indian restaurant an excellent green-light dining option.

There are, however, a few problems to watch out for. The first is that the food is often fried. To make things worse, the food is often fried in 'ghee', or clarified butter, a highly saturated fat. Be sure to ask your waiter how the food is prepared. Choose dishes that are baked or grilled.

The second problem is that full-fat dairy products are sometimes used. Try to avoid dishes with creamy sauces. And avoid bread, which is often made with ghee. If you really, really want bread, choose baked wholemeal chapatti. But it is better to have basmati rice instead. Don't have both.

Many restaurants offer their patrons heaped dishes of coconut slices, raisins and other sweeteners. These are red light. Similarly, be careful of the addition of mangoes and papayas, which are yellow light, in dishes. Guavas are green light.

INDIAN
Butter chicken
Chicken biryani
Chicken korma
Chicken tikka
masala
Curries with
cream sauces
Lamb rogan josh
Naan
Pakoras

INDIAN
Baked chapatti
Prawns madras

INDIAN
Balti vegetables
Bengan bharta
Chicken or fish saag
Chicken tikka
Chicken tikka kebab
Chicken vindaloo
Dal
Fish kebab
Grilled fish
Lentil or bean
dishes without
cream sauces
Steamed basmati rice
Tandoori chicken
or fish
Vegetable curries
without cream
sauces

85

MEXICAN/LATIN AMERICAN

Tex-Mex dishes that are heavy on cheese, refried beans, sour cream and tortillas are unsurprisingly red light. Most 'blackened' dishes are pan-fried in garlic butter and so must be avoided as well. Look for grilled seafood, chicken or meat with salsa, or dishes made with beans (not refried). Gazpacho soups made with tomatoes and peppers are excellent, as is ceviche, which is a seafood dish prepared with citrus juices.

MEXICAN
Burritos
Chorizo
Nachos
Quesadillas

MEXICAN
Chicken fajitas
without the cheese
and sour cream
Chicken or vegetable
enchiladas with red
sauce or salsa
Chilli with beans
and meat

MEXICAN
Arroz abanda
(fish with rice)
Baked fish
Bean and
vegetable soups
Ceviche
Chilli with beans
Chilli with chicken
and beans
Gazpacho
Grilled fish

THAI

Green-light eating is a challenge in Thai restaurants. In the West they tend to rely on sauces to create flavour, rather than spices and herbs as they do in Thailand. Many sauces are very sweet: tamarind sauce, Thai basil sauce and oyster sauce are all red light. Pad Thai, probably the most popular dish, is made with tamarind sauce and rice noodles. Curry sauces and peanut sauce are usually made with full-fat coconut milk and should be avoided, too. 'OK,' you must be thinking, 'is there anything I can eat in a Thai restaurant?'

Yes, actually. Start with a lemongrass soup (without coconut milk!) or mussels in a lemongrass broth. Then have a Thai beef salad, or a stir-fry with chicken and vegetables. Many Thai stir-fries are cooked quickly in small amounts of oil. Satays are also an excellent choice, but skip the peanut sauce. Have your satay with steamed or stir-fried vegetables and a green mango or papaya salad for a fabulous Thai meal.

THAI

Curries containing
coconut milk
Fried rice noodles
Fried spring rolls
Pad Thai
Soups containing
coconut milk

THAI

Cold rolls
(watch the dips)
Green mango salad
(dressing on the side)
Papaya salads

THAI

Chicken or
beef satays
Hot and sour soup
Seafood or
vegetable
soup without
coconut milk
Steamed seafood
Thai beef or chicken
salad (dressing
on side)
Vegetables stir-fried
with little oil

JAPANESE

There are lots of wonderful green-light options at Japanese restaurants once you get beyond the sushi and tempura. Sushi is red light because of the glutinous rice it is made with. Order sashimi instead, which is the fish without the rice. Watch the quantity of soy sauce you use – it's very high in sodium and should be thought of as liquid salt. Other Japanese specialities include wonderful soups made with clear broth bases, sukiyaki, which is a beef and vegetable stir-fry that uses a minimal amount of vegetable oil, and grilled fish. In many restaurants you can prepare your meal yourself in your own group. Nabemono is like a healthy fondue. Into the pot of boiling broth go chunks of vegetables, seafood and so on. Not only is it delicious, but it's also a great experience to share with friends. Miso soup is an excellent source of protein and in Japan it is eaten at the end of the meal to aid digestion.

JAPANESE

Agemono
(deep fried)
Beef teriyaki
Deep fried
pork dishes
Gyoza (fried
dumplings)
Oyako-donburi
(chicken omelette
on rice)
Sushi
Tempura

JAPANESE

Chicken teriyaki
Noodle soup
Pickled salads
Shabu-shabu
Udon

JAPANESE

Grilled seafood
Miso soup
Nabemono
(seafood and
vegetables in
a broth)
Sashimi
Soba
Steamed rice
and vegetables
Stir-fried vegetables
Sukiyaki
Sumashi wan
(clear soup with
tofu and shrimp)
Steamed rice
and vegetables
Yosenabe
(casseroles)

Index